FAMILIES IN THE
REHAB CENTER
AND BEYOND

FAMILIES IN THE REHAB CENTER AND BEYOND

A Survival Guide

DR. MELANIE McCORMICK TIDMAN

Library of Congress Control Number: 2017901388
ISBN: Hardcover   978-1-5245-7912-8
                 Softcover   978-1-5245-7911-1
                 eBook   978-1-5245-7910-4

Print information available on the last page.

Rev. date: 01/27/2017

To order additional copies of this book, contact:
Xlibris
1-888-795-4274
www.Xlibris.com
Orders@Xlibris.com
753896

CONTENTS

DEDICATION

This book is dedicated to my incredible mom who suffered years of health problems and numerous hospitalizations and rehabilitation admissions. It was the issues she faced, the hospitals and rehab centers she was admitted to that were my classroom. I learned not only how to be a daughter helping to support my mother through rehab but also gained knowledge as a professional working with patients and families for over thirty-seven years. I pass onto my families and patients the same information I used with my mom that you will find in this book. I hope this book is a helpful guide for patients and families in transitioning home after an illness or injury. The book was created as part of my mom's legacy. I pray that this book will be an inspiration, resource, and valuable tool for families facing chronic illness, hospitalizations, and loved ones in rehabilitation.

FROM THE AUTHOR. . .

This book is a sequel to my first book entitled *Families in the ICU: A Survival Guide.* This book was developed from a growing concern that families were lacking critical information to assist them while their family member is in a rehabilitation center. I personally have a burden for families when attempting to transition their loved one from rehab to home, and the tremendous stress this places on the family structure, relationships, and on the patient.

I too have lived through this with my mother. Transitions from hospital to rehab to home were difficult until I began to compile this kind of information. Even though I am "in the business" so to speak, I too needed information compiled into one book that I could use as a quick reference guide. I have used this book, in booklet form, with my own patients and their families for many years.

The book is broken up into chapters, and there are places for making notes after each chapter, just as in my first book. None of the information contained in this book is my creation. I have given credit to websites, organizations, and authors. My efforts in creating this book were to merely compile information into one resource, making it more easily accessible to you, the family.

My hope is that this book will provide needed information regarding resources and answer important questions for you, the family, while your loved one is receiving rehabilitation and preparing to return home.
Blessings for good health,

Dr. Melanie McCormick Tidman DHSc, MA, OTR/L

CHAPTER 1

REHAB PERSONNEL ROLES AND RESPONSIBILITIES

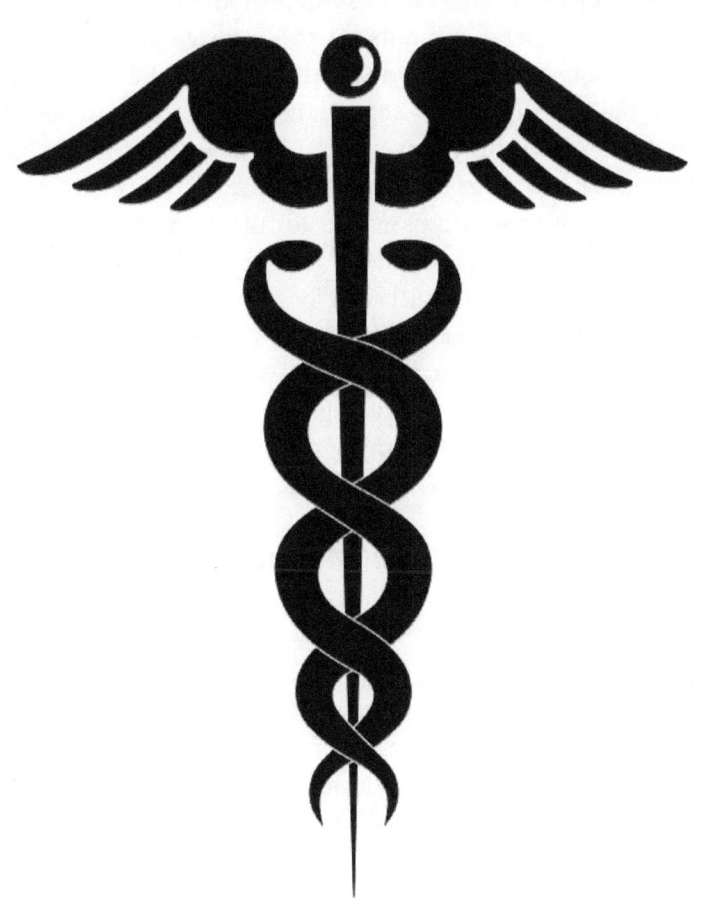

The Admissions Coordinator

You will meet this person while your loved one is still in the hospital. The hospital discharge planner/social worker will provide you with a list of facilities (either skilled rehab or acute rehab) for you to choose one. Once you have made your choice, or taken the recommendations from the social worker/discharge planner, this person will contact the rehab center admissions coordinator. You will then have the opportunity to meet the admissions coordinator, and this person will evaluate your loved one for suitability for rehab. Once this is established, your loved one will be transferred to the rehab center, often by the van provided by the center. You will not need to make any arrangements for the transfer other than to pack up your loved one's personal items and make sure they get to the new center. You also will want to set up and organized your loved one's personal items, labeling everything! Clothes, shoes, socks, and all other personal items with first and last name. This is critical to avoid misplacing any of these items while admitted for rehab in the new center. All of these arrangements should be made automatically, and the admissions coordinator will be responsible for providing you with all needed information, insurance coverage information, a tour of the receiving facility, and acquainting you with the program provided at the new center. Any questions regarding your stay and admission can be directed to the admissions coordinator.

The Social Worker/Case Manager/ Discharge Planner

This is the person who will coordinate with your insurance company during your stay, answer any questions regarding coverage, provide you with information on home health agencies, lead a team meeting with the medical personnel and you, the family, and the patient on a weekly basis to update progress and coordinate your discharge from the facility. This person is a valuable resource for any question regarding these matters.

The Director of Rehabilitation (DOR)

This person directs all aspects of the rehabilitation program and oversees the therapists at the center. He/she is the "go to" person for all questions regarding your loved one's progress, goals, discharge plans for continued rehabilitation, equipment needs, and coordinating family training. Be sure to meet this person when you are first admitted to the center. If you wish to speak with the therapists treating your family member, coordinate with the DOR.

The Physical Therapist (PT)
(http://www.apta.org/AboutPTAs/)

Physical therapists (PTs) are highly educated, licensed health care professionals who can help patients reduce pain and improve or restore mobility—in many cases without expensive surgery and often reducing the need for long-term use of prescription medications and their side effects.

Physical therapists can teach patients how to prevent or manage their condition so that they will achieve long-term health benefits. PTs examine each individual and develop a plan using treatment techniques to promote the ability to move, reduce pain, restore function, and prevent disability. In addition, PTs work with individuals to prevent the loss of mobility before it occurs by developing fitness- and wellness-oriented programs for healthier and more active lifestyles.

Physical therapists provide care for people in a variety of settings, including hospitals, private practices, outpatient clinics, home health agencies, schools, sports and fitness facilities, work settings, and nursing homes. State licensure is required in each state in which a physical therapist practices.

The Physical Therapist Assistant (PTA)
(http://www.apta.org/AboutPTAs/)

Physical therapist assistants (PTAs) provide physical therapy services under the direction and supervision of a licensed physical therapist. PTAs help people of all ages who have medical problems or other health-related conditions that limit their ability to move and perform functional activities in their daily lives. PTAs may also measure changes in the patient's performance as a result of the physical therapy provided.

Care provided by a PTA may include teaching patients/clients exercise for mobility, strength and coordination, training for activities such as walking with crutches, canes, or walkers, massage, and the use of physical agents and electrotherapy such as ultrasound and electrical stimulation.

The Occupational Therapist (OT)
(http://www.aota.org/About-Occupational-Therapy/Professionals. aspx#sthash.u3F47C85.dpuf)

Occupational therapists (OT) and occupational therapist assistants (OTA) help people of all ages participate in the things they want and need to do through the therapeutic use of everyday activities (occupations). Unlike other professions, occupational therapy helps people function in all of their environments (e.g., home, work, school, community) and addresses the physical, psychological, and cognitive aspects of their well-being through engagement in occupation.

Occupational therapy services typically include:

- an individualized evaluation during which the client, family, and occupational therapist determine the person's goals,
- customized intervention to improve the person's ability to perform daily activities and reach the goals, and
- an outcome evaluation to ensure that the goals are being met and/or to modify the intervention plan based on the patient's needs and skills.

Occupational therapy services may include comprehensive evaluations of the client's home and other environments, recommendations for adaptive equipment and training in its use, training in how to modify a task or activity to facilitate participation, and guidance and education for family members and caregivers. Entry-level practice requires a master's degree for occupational therapists and an associate's degree for occupational therapist assistants (who must be supervised by an OT).(See more at http://www.aota.org/About-Occupational-Therapy/Professionals.aspx#sthash.u3F47C85.dpuf)

The Speech Language Pathologist
(http://www.asha.org/careers/recruitment/healthcare/)

Speech language pathologists (SLPs) are essential professionals in every health care setting—acute care, rehabilitation, pediatric, and psychiatric hospitals, long-term care, outpatient facilities, and home health. Their expertise provides invaluable benefit to patients and other staff in managing problems (swallowing, communication, and cognitive linguistic disorders) that affect patients' overall health, well-being, and ability to benefit from other medical or rehabilitation interventions.

The Rehab Doctor: Physiatrist
(https://www.aapmr.org/patients/aboutpmr/Pages/physiatrist.aspx)

Physiatrists, or rehabilitation physicians, are nerve, muscle, and bone experts who treat injuries or illnesses that affect how you move. Rehabilitation physicians are medical doctors who have completed training in the medical specialty of physical medicine and rehabilitation (PM&R). Specifically, rehabilitation physicians:

- Diagnose and treat pain
- Restore maximum function lost through injury, illness, or disabling conditions
- Treat the whole person, not just the problem area
- Lead a team of medical professionals
- Provide nonsurgical treatments
- Explain your medical problems and treatment/prevention plan

The job of a rehabilitation physician is to treat any disability resulting from disease or injury, from sore shoulders to spinal cord injuries. The focus is on the development of a comprehensive program for putting the pieces of a person's life back together after injury or disease—without surgery.

Director of Nursing and Assistant Director of Nursing

This person is a nursing department director and oversees the function of the nursing staff including RNs and CNAs. This may be a good person to speak with if there are any issues with nursing while your loved one is in rehab.

The Nurse
(http://everydaylife.globalpost.com/role-registered-nurse-skilled-facility-18341.html)

A skilled nursing facility also called a nursing home or long-term care facility caters to patients who require around-the-clock care. This includes everyone from elderly patients to those with chronic or degenerative conditions and those recovering from traumatic injury or illness. While certified nursing assistants and licensed practical nurses provide much of the day-to-day care in these facilities, registered nurses play a crucial role in overseeing treatment and ensuring all patients receive the highest standard of care.

LPNs and CNAs are limited in the kinds of tasks they can perform, so RNs perform much of the more complex or invasive treatment. For example, they administer medications and injections, take blood, and prepare and insert IV lines. They also monitor each patient's health and progress by evaluating his vital signs and assessing other indications of his physical and mental well-being. In addition, they determine the treatment plan for each patient and ensure the care strategy addresses the long-term needs of the aging process and the conditions with which he's coping.

Certified Nursing Assistants

These people are the ones your loved one will see most often. They are responsible for all aspects of bedside care including assistance with toileting, dressing, and hygiene, grooming, getting patients out of bed in the morning and ready for rehab, and assisting patients to meals. They check vital signs on a variable schedule (some patients are checked every shift, some each day, and some once a week depending on the doctor's orders), and then tuck your loved one back into bed at the end of the day. CNAs are trained, frequently, by OT and PT regarding transfer safety and care for mobility and self-care needs of the patient.

Certified Medication Assistant

In the hospital, you may have been used to a nurse providing medications to your loved one. In rehab, a certified medication tech, especially at the skilled rehab level and in the long-term care center, administers medications. CMAs are supervised by RNs. Medications in acute rehab are still administered by an RN or LPN.

The Dietitian

This person is an expert in nutrition and evaluates the nutritional needs of your loved one along with nursing and the doctor in charge. The dietitian will make recommendations for balancing nutrients and overseeing general dietary needs while your loved one is in rehab. This person is specifically knowledgeable about tube feedings or supplemental feedings if needed.

Kitchen Manager

This person is responsible for the running of the kitchen, tray set up and dissemination, snacks, etc. The kitchen manager also coordinates with the dietitian on meal orders for patients and feeding recommendations from occupational and speech therapy. Any needed equipment or adaptations for feeding should be address to the kitchen manager.

Activities Director

This person is responsible for the extracurricular activities that occur in the rehab center outside of therapy. This is a program most often offered in the skilled rehab center and long-term care facility. Some acute care rehab centers offer an activity programs but not as many have this as those patients spending more time in therapy than in the skilled rehab center.

This person can also help coordinate special parties for your loved one with you for birthdays or other special occasions. There is a daily activity schedule usually posted or printed out for you and your loved one, and your loved one is highly encouraged to participate in as many activities as possible. It is participation in the therapy program along with participation in extra activities that builds strength, endurance, and maintains social interaction while in the rehab center.

Administrator

This is the "Big Boss" of the rehab facility. This person oversees all areas of the facility with input from all department directors and managers. If your concerns have not been addressed to your satisfaction with specific departmental directors, you may want to make an appointment with the administrator.

Medical Records

It is highly suggested that you meet these folks to obtain a release of information form for your loved one to sign, so you may receive all documents associated with the rehab stay, records from therapy, medical records, etc. These records are crucial to provide to your loved one's primary care physician upon discharging, so he/she has a record of what occurred while in rehab.

The Billing Office

This department is responsible for billing any extra charges to you, the family, or to the patient. It is a good idea to check with these folks as to any outstanding balance that may be due. Also, many facilities have a patient account that you can set up so your loved one can take advantage of the salon services (haircuts, nails done, etc.). These services are done by appointment only, and you will need to contact the salon itself. Typically, contact information is placed on the door of the salon. You may call and set up appointments for your loved one. These services are on a self-pay basis. The facility does not pay for these extra services.

The State Ombudsman (Look for the Aging and Long Term services department in your state)

Ombudsman services are available in all states, and the word ombudsman means "citizen's representative." This is a person whose job is to protect the rights of patients using long-term services and encourage facility to also uphold and respect those rights. Ombudsman services are usually run by volunteers who visit patients in nursing homes, assisted living, and long-term nursing facilities. Their duty is to assist residents and patients/families in voicing their concerns and seeking way to address their concerns when usual methods have not brought resolution. They serve as mediators between patients/families and facility administrations to improve both quality of life and quality of care for those patients who live in either long-term care facilities or are admitted for rehabilitation. Their role is to advocate, educate, investigate, collaborate, empower, visit, mediate, and respect the needs of patients/families to bring about positive results.

The Insurance Company Nurse Case Manager

This person is typically an RN who is employed by your insurance company to check on your progress and program in the rehab center and coordinate care with the insurance company. This person will be knowledgeable about your benefits and the length of stay and services that will be reimbursed by your insurance company. This person is crucial in deciding when your loved one will be discharged and when insurance coverage for the stay will end. Typically, this person meets with the rehab and nursing team on a weekly basis to discuss patient's progress and possible discharge dates.

NOTES

CHAPTER 2

COMMON TERMINOLOGY
IN THE REHABILITATION CENTER

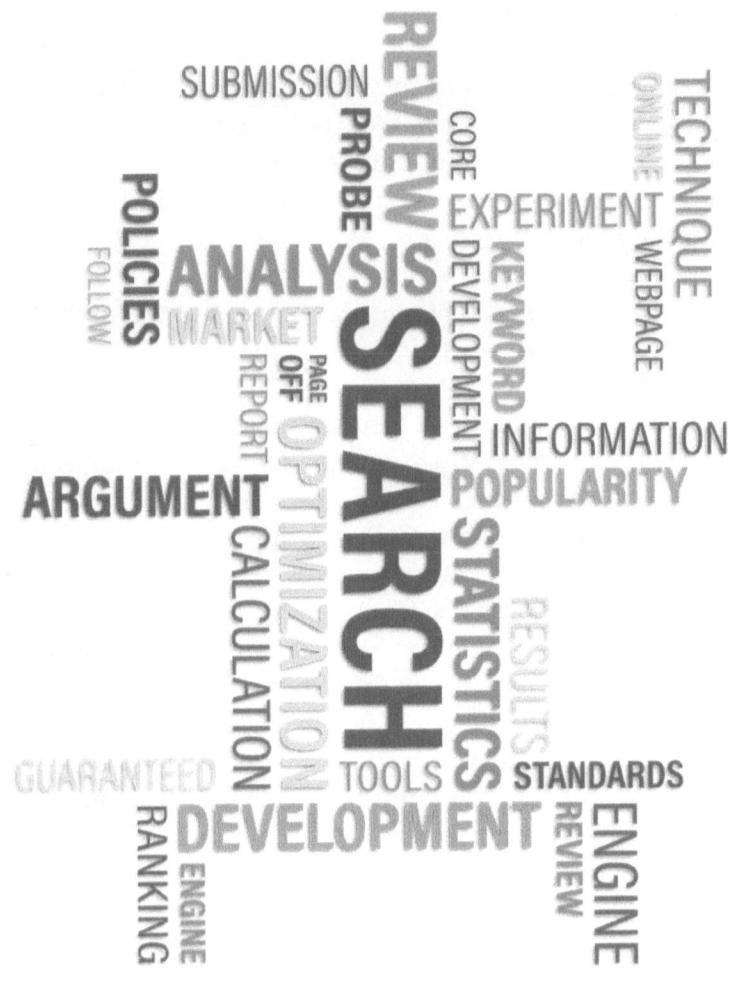

Acute Rehabilitation

Rehabilitation including occupational, physical, and speech therapy services on an intensive basis with therapy participation expectations at three to five hours per day. Be sure your loved one can participate at this level prior to discharge to this intensity of rehab. There are other options available for rehab that require less participation time per day. Double-check your loved one's ability to participate at this level with the therapists.

Admission Paperwork Terminology
Code Terminology

There are various code words that the rehab staff uses to communicate with each other. Generally, you do not have to know these as they affect main communication between the staff at the facility. Hospitals also use some of these code words. Here are a few most common ones:

- Code Red: indicates there is a fire in some part of the facility. You will hear instructions as to what you need to do in the event of a fire
- Code Blue: indicates a patient is in severe distress, requiring emergency medical treatment, was found unresponsive, or has suffered an even affecting heart functions.
- Code Black: in some facilities, this means there is a utility outage. You will be instructed as to what you need to do.
- Code White: in some facilities, this means a terrorist attack.
- Code Pink: in some facilities, this means a resident cannot be located, and may have left the facility unescorted or unexpectedly. There are some residents who are not aware of the safety, and they may try to walk out with you through an exit door. Check with nursing to see if the patient is allowed to go outside the facility.
- Code Green: there is an impending severe weather event or natural disaster.

Discharge Planning Terminology

- Durable Medical Equipment: see terms and definition in Chapter 5.

The DNR/DNI Consent

This is an important consent form that must be signed by the patient (if pt. has the capacity to make his/her own decisions) or by the power of attorney. The DNR means "Do Not Resuscitate." If the patient has a cardiac arrest, no resuscitation attempts will be made if a DNR consent form has been signed. DNI means do not intubate. This means that the patient is not to be intubated (a breathing tube placed down the throat). These decisions are very important as they make the difference on what treatments will be given should an emergency occur. Please discuss this with your loved one in detail, and let the rehab staff and therapists know what the wishes of the patient are. Then either have them sign or not sign the DNR/DNI form provided by the facility. Many patients decide they do not want to be resuscitated if a major event occurs due to the likelihood that they would not recover and would have to be put through the ordeal of maintaining life support machines until the family make the decision to turn them off. This is a conversation every family must have with the elderly family members to see what it is that they want at the end of their life.

Home Health Care (HHC)

HHC services are arranged by the social worker/discharge planner at the rehab facility just prior to discharge. HHC services generally consist of nursing care (provided once or twice a week to check on patients status), physical therapy (provided two to three times per week as necessary), occupational and speech therapy services (provided as needed but typically not more than two to three times per week or less), and an aide to assist with self-care and bathing (as needed). If the patient requires wound care at home, daily wound care or IV antibiotic management is arranged in some cases. These professionals come to the home. You should be contacted by the HHC nurse shortly after you get home so be aware for this phone call.

Hospice/Palliative Care

These services are provided toward the end of life if patients have a severe terminal condition or if patients and family members want supporting care only. Often these services involve nursing care and comfort care services. These services are mainly provided to patients who will not recover but wish to have supportive care and adequate pain control toward the end of their lives. These services can be provided in a long-term care facility at home or in a special hospice inpatient facility.

Long-Term Care:

These services are provided when patients and/or families can no longer care for the individual in a home setting. Patients then live in a Long-Term Care (LTC) facility where meals and self-care are provided. LTCs are for patients who are unable to care for themselves and require assistance for most self-care tasks (toileting, dressing, bathing, etc.). Limited therapy services may be available through the patient's Medicare Part B coverage. Check with the social worker in the facility to see if your loved one qualifies. Mainly, these therapists are provided 3x/wk.

Medication Management Terminology

Scheduled Medications: These are routine medications that are scheduled to be given to your loved one at specific times during the day. Check with the certified medication assistant to see what this schedule is.

PRN Medications: PRN means "on call" or "on request." This means your loved one will have to request these medications as needed. This is very common for pain medications. In the hospital, these may have been scheduled medications to help control the early pain symptoms. Now that your loved one is in rehab, these medications become "on request" as the pain should be under control. Encourage your loved one to request pain medications before the pain becomes unbearable. Keep in mind that most pain medications need twenty to thirty minutes to become effective. Don't wait! If your loved one's pain is not well controlled over a few days and the pain interferes with the rehabilitation, speak with the nurse (not the CMA) regarding either a change in medication or placing pain medications on a scheduled basis for a few days to get the pain under control. It is important that pain should not interfere with the rehabilitation process and that your loved one receives as much therapy as possible while in the rehab center. The nurse and the facility physician will work with pain medications to insure the pain is tolerable, perhaps not gone all together but tolerable to allow for therapy participation.

The NOC Letter

This letter will be given to you and your loved one at least forty-eight to seventy-two hours prior to discharge. This is a letter that is required by Medicare regulations to inform you of the discharge date. Your social worker can explain the letter further to your understanding. Keep in mind that you have the right to appeal any discharge that you feel is too soon, or if you feel strongly that your loved one needs more therapy. Review patient's rights on a document that the facility should have provided you when your loved one was admitted to the facility.

Pain Scores/Grading Your Pain

The Visual Analog Scale: A pain scales from one to ten used to analyze a patient's pain in order to provide pain medication. A score of one is no pain at all up to ten which is the worst pain imaginable. Most patients have difficulty providing a pain score, and will need your assistance in determining just how bad their pain is. Work with your loved one to accurately report their pain level as this will determine just how much and when they receive their pain medication.

The Wong Faces Scale: These are presented to the patient as pictures of different faces illustrating different levels of pain. Patients who are unable to determine a number for their pain or patients who are severely hard of hearing or speaking another language can benefit from use of this pain scale.

Rehabilitation Terminology

Levels of Assistance/Grading Assistance Needed

These levels are decided using scored from the Functional Independence Measure or FIM. FIM scores give everyone an idea of what level of assistance is needed for your loved one to perform certain tasks. These levels serve as a communication tool between rehab personnel to note changes in function, progress, and attainment of goals.

> Independent—Score 7: This score reflects a typical person functioning with anyone around for all tasks that allow him/her to participate in daily living, work, mobility, and transportation, self-care, hygiene, and leisure.

> Modified Independent—Score 6: This score reflects a person who is able to function well without any assistance, but either requires a bit more time to complete tasks, uses any type of assistive device such as a walker, but is completely independent in all needed areas of life skills.

Supervision/Standby Assistance (SPV/SBA)—Score 5: This score reflects someone who is physically capable of all tasks but may require someone to be watching due to issues with balance, safety, or reminders to complete certain tasks.

Contact Guard Assistance—(Score is still 4): This is when only a steadying hand or light touch is required. Otherwise, the loved one can perform all needed tasks.

Minimum Assistance—Score 4: This reflects the need for the assistant to provide approximately 25% of the assistance, where the person performs 75% of the task. Example of this would be holding a coat, so the person can put it on.

Moderate Assistance—Score 3: This level reflects a person who requires 50% assistance to complete tasks with 50% being provided by the assistant.

Maximum Assistance—Score 2: This reflects a person who requires 75% assistance from the assistant and is only able to perform 25% of the task.

Dependent—Score 1: This reflects a person who requires total assistance and cannot participate in any of the task. The assistant must provide 100% of the assistance, which may include totally lifting the person from one place to another. Patients at this level seldom discharge home. Some facilities call this total assistance.

Skilled Rehabilitation

A rehabilitation facility which may include occupational, physical, and speech therapy where participation expectations are two to three hours per day.

Transfers

Moving from one place to another either in seated position or while standing. For example: moving from a bed to a wheelchair, wheelchair to a toilet, standing into a car, standing to sitting, sitting up into a walker, etc.

A Stand Pivot Transfer—while standing, the person pivots feet around to sit in a location (either a chair or bed) placed at a forty-five-degree angle.

A Scoot Pivot Transfer—while seated, the person scoots his/her bottom from one location to another. This transfer does not involve standing but does involve some leg strength and arm strength.

A Sliding Board Transfer—this transfer uses a device called a sliding board which is often a board, approximately 24–32" long, placed under the bottom on one end and on the surface on the other end. The person then scoots along the board to the new location. Assistance is needed in steadying the board on the new location.

A Hoyer Life or Dependent Transfer—this is a mechanical lift device requiring training, a sling to hold the person, and a large, overhead lift. This can be either totally mechanical (crank) or electronic (a control device or button requiring electricity to operate). The rehab staff will need to train you on this device if this is the chosen device for your loved one. Assistance often requires two people.

Types of Rehabilitation Beds

The Hi-Lo Bed: This bed adjusts from a high level for ease of patient turning to the floor for fall prevention. This bed is particularly beneficial for transfers involving a scoot pivot technique (see above). Although it is not usual, these beds can be fitted with bed rails at least on one side for ease of transfers and turning in bed.

> The ERU Bed: This bed is typically higher than a normal bed, have bed rails on both sides for ease of bed mobility, and have positioning adjustments in more positions than a Hi-Lo Bed. These beds may be too high for short patients and typically are too high for the scoot pivot technique (see above) in most cases. If this is the case for your loved one, ask the nurse or Director of Nursing if your loved one can have a Hi-Lo Bed.

> The Air Mattress Bed: These beds are to accommodate an air mattress, usually only ordered for those patients with wounds. Air mattresses used air to vary the pressure throughout the bed for pressure relief.

Types of Rehab Equipment for Mobility:
(common types)

> Front Wheeled Walker (FWW)
> Four Wheeled Walker (4WW)
> Single Point Cane (SPC)
> Quad Cane (QC)
> Hemi-Walker

> Platform Walker: like a standard FWW but has a platform on either one or both sides where patients rest their forearms. These are specifically effective for patients who have extremely weak legs and arms.

The patient bears weight through the entire forearm to assist with walking in the walker.

Wheelchair: Manual Mobility (W/C)
Reclining High Back
Non-Reclining Standard Back wheelchair

One-Handed Propulsion Assist: this type of wheelchair is specifically helpful for those patients who have suffered a stroke and have little or no use of one arm or leg on one side of their body.

Wheelchair: Powered Mobility (PW/C)

Wound Care Terminology:

The RN in the rehab center typically oversees the wound care. The doctor will order the wound care regimen that is needed, and the RN carries this through. In many rehab centers, either occupational or physical therapists also assist with wound care.

What is a Wound Vac? This is a device placed on some wounds to encourage healing. This device is usually used for deep wounds or wounds that have not healed. Think of this machine as a vacuum that is placed on the wound to draw the circulation to the surface and help to heal the wound. The device is attached to the wound by a long tube, which will then be attached to a small machine that applies suction. The RN will check the device and oversee use and changing of the wound vac and dressings. Ask the RN what the schedule for wound care is (daily, every other day, etc.)

Stages of Wounds

Stage 1—Wounds do not have skin tears or cuts that are visible. The skin covering the wound looks different than the surrounding skin and maybe red, warm to the touch, or either softer/harder than normal skin.

Stage II—The topmost layers of the skin are affected and maybe open with some drainage.

Stage III—These wounds are deeper and go down to the fat layer. There is dead tissue visible and drainage.

Stage IV—These wounds are very serious and may go as deep as the bone with dead tissue and drainage.

Signs and symptoms of wounds that you should tell the nurse about are wounds with pus or drainage of any kinds, redness, and swelling with warmth on or around the wound, increased pain, bleeding, fever, no healing in ten days or longer, and/or numbness.

NOTES

CHAPTER 3

THE DISCHARGE PLANNING AND FAMILY/TEAM MEETING PROCESS

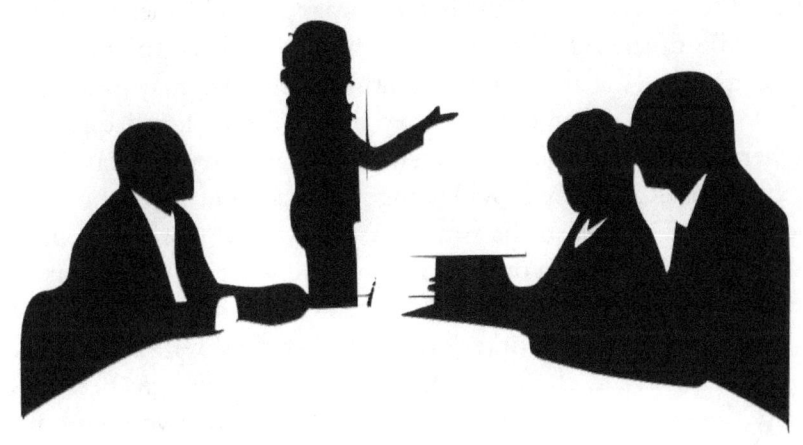

Meeting Notification

You and your loved one will be notified of a team meeting scheduled with you, your loved one, the facility social worker, Director of Nursing, Director of Rehabilitation, kitchen manager, or dietitian (in some cases), insurance nurse (representing your insurance company),treating therapists, and the person at the facility in charge of billing processes (in some cases). You have the right to have anyone present at this meeting that you choose including a request for the therapists who have been working with your loved one to be present (in most cases). Frequently, the facility physician will attend these meetings but not always. You may request the facility physician be present to address specific medical concerns that you feel the nursing staff may not be able to address.

The team meeting is the time to ask questions about medications, medical tests needed, recent therapy progress, any issues of medical care while in the rehab center, and discharge plans. In addition to discharge plans, ask about home health agencies that may be available to help you and what services they offer. If your loved one needs further therapy, the team may recommend an extended stay or that the home health agency provides ongoing treatment when the patient goes home. This is also the time to ask the social worker about any discharge equipment recommendations, and whether your insurance will cover the cost of purchasing these items, whether they will be ordered by the social worker, and whether they will be delivered to your home or to the rehab center prior to discharge. Be sure to clarify this so you have the needed equipment when you get home. The therapists should have discussed what was needed with you at some point in the rehab program.

These meetings are important and are typically scheduled once a week or as needed. You may request a team meeting at any time. If you have not had a team meeting and want one, please contact your facility social worker/discharge planner to schedule one.

NOTES

CHAPTER 4

HOME SAFETY ASSESSMENT

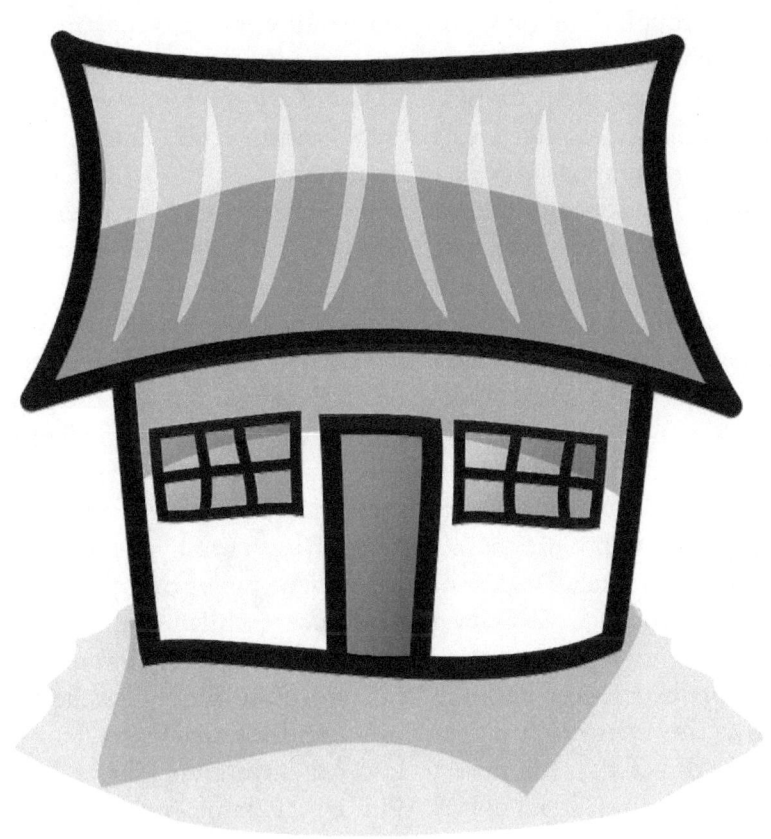

Setting: A home safety and equipment assessment includes the location of the patient's home, neighborhood environment, street access, entry steps if any, access to public transportation, any neighborhood covenants that must be followed, family structure and availability of assistance from family members, and access to transportation.

Barriers: Walk around your house and list any access barriers. I recommend walking around the house with whatever device your family member will be using once they go home. If the patient will be using a front wheeled walker (FWW), borrow one and walk with it through doorways, around furniture, etc. Do the same with a wheelchair (W/C). Make note of those places where access is restricted. Make plans to move furniture around to allow for easier access inside the house. Using a tape measure, take measurements of all door openings, measure doorways both inside and outside including interior and exterior doors. A standard door opening to accommodate most wheelchairs needs to be at least thirty-two inches measured from inside the doorjamb.

Kitchen: Furniture or small appliances may need to be moved to allow the patient to access the kitchen area including kitchen sink, microwave, stove, cabinets, and refrigerator. Be sure the patient can access from either the FWW (if that is the chosen device) or a wheelchair (if the plan is to use this when discharged). Make sure the patient can adequately reach the microwave for cooking, and suggest to the patient to not use the stove to cook with until you are sure he/she can do so safely. Make sure the patient can turn light switches on and off from the W/C level or can access while using the FWW. Moving about without proper lighting can be a safety hazard.

Bedroom: Most patients' beds are quite high. I suggest you remove the mattress from its frame, and set the box spring and mattress directly on the floor to lower the overall height of the bed for ease of getting in/out of bed. Without the frame, most patients can demonstrate a scoot pivot transfer from the W/C to the bed and from the bed to the W/C with improved safety. Family members should be trained on this transfer prior to leaving the rehab center. I suggest you to purchase a portable bed rail, easily installed on the entry/exit side of the bed. Borrow/Rent/Buy a bedside commode for placement beside the bed for ease and safety of nighttime bathroom visits (see

Chapter 5 for Durable Medical Equipment). Bedsides commodes work best using the bariatric style with bilateral platforms, drop arms, and adjustable height. The patient and the family should be trained to safely perform bedside commode transfers prior to leaving the rehab center by occupational therapy. If this has not been done, ask the occupational therapist prior to discharge.

Bathroom: Bathroom equipment is essential and, in some cases, much cheaper and less time consuming than hiring someone to renovate the bathroom. Often installing all needed grab bars is the most difficult. Try contacting the Department of Senior Affairs in your city to see if they install grab bars as a community service. This service is free in most cases. Obtaining needed equipment needs to occur before the patient comes home.

I recommend family members to ask the occupational and physical therapists what equipment is anticipated at least one week prior to the planned discharge date. Common bathroom adaptations include a tub transfer bench with built-in grab bar, a handheld showerhead, and a toilet safety frame (See Chapter 5). Once again, check the access to the tub using the W/C or FWW. Families should be trained on safe transfer techniques in the bathroom by the occupational therapist. Be sure to obtain this training prior to discharge. Be sure the patient can access the sink while seated in the W/C. This is often a problem. Alternative would be to have a basin the patient can use for toothbrushing set near the sink. This basin can be held in the patient's lap and toothbrushing and face washing can be performed without having to stretch to reach the sink from a seated position. Bathroom doorways are often not wide enough. If only 1–1 ½" is lacking, obtain and install easy access door hinges (also called swing away door hinges) which provide 1–2" more clearance. Most medical supply stores have these, and only a screwdriver is needed to install them (see Chapter 5).

Garden/Yard Area: If the patient has outdoor activities he/she enjoys, evaluate garden/yard area access. Ask yourself, "Are the sidewalks and driveways of adequate width and slope can accommodate a W/C or FWW safely?" "Can the patient get out the front door, down a narrow sidewalk, around the corner, and move about in the yard?" I suggest you raise garden activities to W/C level by placing things in pots on a table surface or building raised gardening frames where the W/C can slide under for ease of reach. Raised garden beds built up on tabletop surfaces also can accommodate the W/C. It is important that the patient will be able to resume activities for enjoyment as soon as they are able. A good idea is to give no access to the patient on the garden initially without a family member present.

General Safety Considerations: Remove all throw rugs and loose carpeting that could cause the patient to trip. Walk through the house with the device the patient will be using (such as a walker) to see if the device fits through doorways. Watch for electrical cords stretched across the floor where the patient can trip and fall. Widen doorways as much as possible, and often it is helpful to remove a door all together to allow for easier access with a walker or wheelchair. Remove clutter! Less furniture is much safer than rooms crammed with furniture. Widen walking pathways to at least thirty-two inches. You may need to rearrange furniture or get rid of furniture to allow for more room for mobility around the house.

Remove glass shower doors and replace with a shower curtain for ease of using a tub transfer bench for access to the tub or shower. Glass doors may shatter if the patient falls. Install grab bars in the shower if possible. Many options for grab bars are found at local Do-It-Yourself stores. Purchase a rubber suction mat for inside the shower and (if the floor is flooring and not carpeted) outside the shower. This will provide a nonskid surface inside the shower and outside as well. The patient should never stand up in the shower. Sitting while in the shower is much safer. Always have them shower when someone else is at the home for safety reasons.

Pill minders make medication administration much safer. A family member may need to set up the pill boxes ahead of time. Medication errors are the most common reason an elderly person is admitted to the hospital.

Subscribe to a Lifeline or Life Alert monitoring system that provides a necklace/button to your family member that they can push when they fall or need assistance. These services are inexpensive and well worth it if you will not be able to be with your loved one 24/7. Contact your local EMS and ask them about setting up a lockbox with a key that they can access should they need to get to your loved one quickly. This way, they won't need to break the door down or break through a window. They will be the only ones with access to this key much like Realtors do when they are showing a home to prospective clients. These monitoring services will call you first, if you put your contact information on the list, when they receive an alert to ask you to check on your loved one.

Summary and Equipment List: Summarize your list and access issues. Make a plan to talk with the occupational or physical therapist regarding ideas to adapt daily living task issues and find solutions to these issues at least one week prior to discharge. Another recommendation is to obtain a home monitoring service like Lifeline or Life Alert for safety monitoring if patient is to be alone at times during the day or night once they are home. Use of baby monitors placed throughout the home is also recommended for patients to contact the caregiver if they were in a different part of the house. An important suggestion is to contact the local EMS station to set up a lockbox monitoring system for EMS to safety and quickly access patient's home if patient will be alone. EMS will be the only ones with the code to open the lockbox and access a key to get into the home should patient require medical assistance. Otherwise, they will need to break a window or door to enter the home. This saves costs to repair/replace doors or windows.

Transportation for both medical and nonmedical assistance to help the patient transport to medical and nonmedical appointments is also recommended. Most patients will require assistance in transporting via a W/C. The physical therapist will need to review safety with the family, and train techniques for safe car transfers prior to discharge.

NOTES

CHAPTER 5

DURABLE MEDICAL EQUIPMENT AND HOME MODIFICATIONS

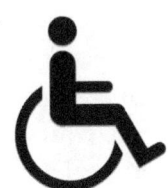

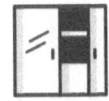 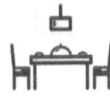

 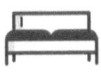

 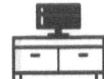 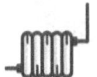

 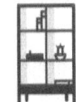 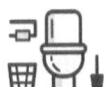

    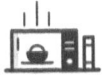

Wheelchair Prescription

The physical and/or occupational therapist are responsible for informing you, the patient, and the social worker/discharge planner about the requirements for a wheelchair. This wheelchair will be fitted to specifications that the therapists feel are important for the safety and mobility of your loved one once he/she is discharged home. Typically, wheelchairs have the following options available:

Removable Desk Arms: A must for ease of transfers and positioning at a table.

Removable Foot Rests either standard or elevating: Standard footrests are fine for most patients. Elevating foot rests are for patients who have chronic swelling (we call it edema) in their legs, feet, or ankles. The elevating leg rests can be periodically elevated during the day to help bring down leg/ankle swelling.

Standard Back versus High Back: Standard back height is typical for most people. A high back wheelchair is needed for those patients who have poor head control and need extra support to position their head/neck.

Reclining versus Standard Wheelchair: Some chairs have a high back that reclines which is helpful for pressure relief and positioning during the day. Other chairs have what is called a "tilt-in-space" feature where the seat back and seat bottom recline as a unit, placing the patient in a fully reclined position. This position is helpful for patients who have chronic wounds on their bottom who need pressure relief throughout the day and cannot perform this repositioning themselves.

Bathroom Equipment

Toilet Safety Frame
Toilet Riser
Shower Chair with Back and Arms
Handheld Shower Wand
Grab Bars for Shower, Tub, or Toilet
Bedside Commode

Easy Access Door Hinges: You can replace regular door hinges with these, and the door will swing away and lay flat against the wall giving as much as 1–1 ½" more clearance for wheelchairs or walkers to fit through the door. These can be bought at a medical equipment supply and typically cost between $30 and $40. To install, you will need a screwdriver.

Tub Transfer Bench: A special bench for the bathtub where one half of the bench sits inside the tub and one half sits outside the tub on the floor. The patient sits down on the bench and slides across into the tub, lifting both legs into the tub. This prevents the patient from needing to step in/out of the tub, which can be very dangerous. Also, because the patient is seated for the entire process of showering, you do not need to install expensive grab bars in the shower/tub area which can be costly and, in some cases, not possible. The patient should never stand in the bathtub but stay seated and perform all showering. Be sure you install a handheld shower wand with the tub transfer bench, so the patient can shower while seated and control the water.

Ramps and Access Issues
Websites for portable step ramps:
Van Ramps (portable)

Kitchen Issues and Modifications

> Resources for adaptive feeding and cooking equipment: catalogs include Sammons Preston, Invacare, and other special DME catalogs and websites.

> Examples of adaptive feeding equipment include a plate guard (to keep food from falling off the plate and give the patient something to scoop against), large handled utensils (for ease of grasp), universal cuff (a cuff that holds spoons or forks for patients whose grasp is too weak to hold utensils). All the patient does is bring the food to his/her mouth. The cuff grips the utensil. These are also helpful for toothbrushes and rattail combs/picks. Consult the OT for one of these.

Low Vision Modifications

Resources for low vision evaluation and training: In many cases, training is provided by the Commission for the Blind in your state. Go to the State Department of Health and Human Services website for information on these services. Modifications can be as simple as placing bright fluorescent green or yellow duct tape on items the patient needs to grasp or reach for (such as call lights, bed rails, wheelchair arms, and grab bars). The concept is to try to mark objects with high contrasting colors (i.e. black on white is the highest contrast and easier to see) to make items easier to locate.

Bedroom Issues and Modifications

Bed Too High: When possible, remove the bed and box spring from the frame and place them on the floor. This lowers the bed by several inches in most cases for ease of getting in/out of bed.

Furniture in the Way: I suggest you to get a walker or wheelchair and move around your loved one's home environment. Note those areas where furniture may need to be moved or rearranged for ease of access.

Doorways Too Narrow: Note how narrow the doorways are and make note of measurements of doorways that must be used by the patient in either a wheelchair or a walker. In some cases, extra space is provided through doorways by installing easy access or swing away door hinges. This will work well if only one inch to one and a half inches are needed for the wheelchair or walkers to get through the door. Much more than this, it probably will not be possible for the patient to access the rooms through these narrow doors without some costly remodeling. If the bathroom is the problem (i.e. wheelchair is too wide to fit through the bathroom door), get a bedside commode, and set it up in a place where the patient can wheel up to it in the wheelchair and transfer on/off the commode. (Helpful hint: bedside commodes can double as shower chairs for walk-in showers. Just remove the bucket!)

Estimated/Approximate Costs for Common Home Equipment
(Of course prices may vary)

This is only an idea of the approximate costs of needed home equipment, often then can be obtained for free from organizations that lend these items. Shop on the internet and at DIY stores for good prices.

Toilet Safety Frames-Standard/Drop Arm	$75.00
Toilet Safety Frames-Bariatric/Drop Arm	$165.00
Bedside Commodes-Standard/Drop Arm	$165.00
Bedside Commodes-Bariatric/Drop Arm	$250.00
Grab Bars for Shower	$35.00
Plate Guards	$8.00
Rocker Knives—to assist patient with cutting food	$18.00
Rojo Cushions-Standard for patients with a pressure ulcer)	$70.00
Lateral W/C Trunk supports (for patients who need help sitting up in wheelchair)	$185.00
Stroke Wheelchair Arm Troughs	$135.00
Incentive Spirometers—for pneumonia	$58.00
Volar Wrist Cock Up Splints—Large	$21.00
ADL Dressing Kits	$20.00
Reachers—32"	$10.00
Dycem—nonslip mat	$45.00/roll

NOTES

CHAPTER 6

SERVICES ONCE YOU ARE HOME

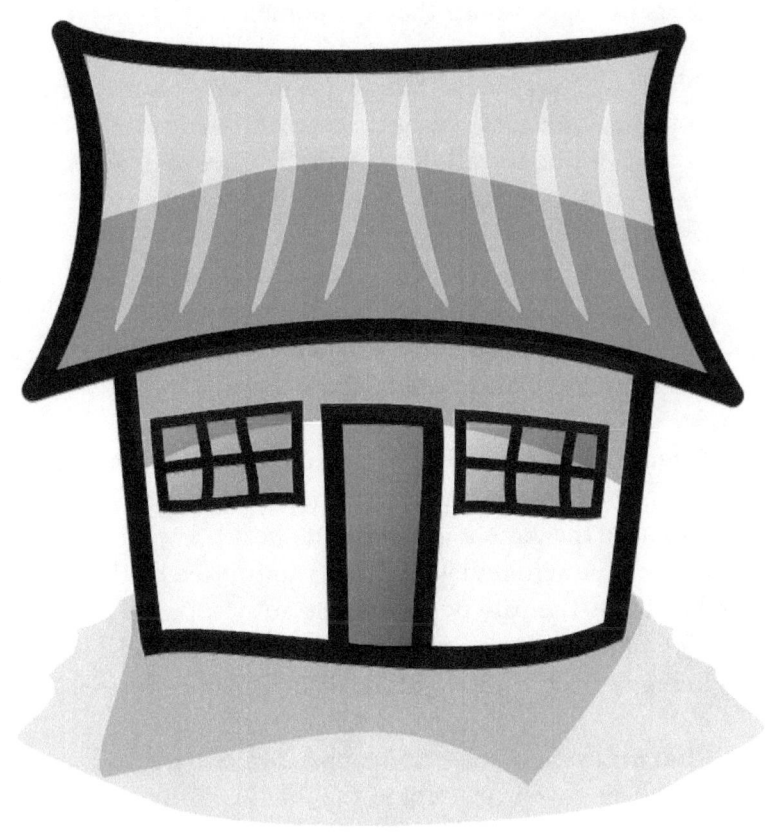

Home Health Care Roles and Responsibilities

The Evaluation: This evaluation includes a review of medications (have your loved one's medication list handy), any wound care needs, medical history, current medical issues, a brief review of the rehab stay, and any needs you may want to bring up such as assistance for bathing or household tasks. The nurse will write up what is called a plan of care which addresses your loved one's specific needs, need for therapy (either PT, OT, or speech), dietary needs, needs for supplies, and any need for follow-up visits to the patient's primary physician (which needs to happen once they get home).

Home Nursing Services: Home health care nurses check in typically once a week to monitor the status of the patient. This can occur as a visit or phone call. Keep a list of questions, so when the nurse calls or visits, you can ask them and get some answers.

Home Health Aide Services: Typically, these services are for bathing and personal care and occur usually around 2x/week. The plan of care designed by the nurse will determine how often the aide comes to assist in these areas and for how long.

Home Telemedicine Services: In many regions, the home health care agency provides a machine to monitor the patient's vital signs, weight, and have the patient answer some health questions. A nurse at a central location will review the data transmitted by this machine daily and call you/the patient if there are any concerns. Ask for this service. Not all home health care agencies have this available, but for patients living in remote areas, this is an extremely important service.

Home Pharmacy Services: Some pharmacies have an automated machine medication service where they deliver a machine already set up with your loved one's medications. The machine dispenses the medications at certain times each day (whatever the doctor prescribed). This is a great service, if offered in your area, for those medications that are routine and taken every day at around the same time. Call your local pharmacy and ask about this service. Otherwise, if you need to set up your loved one's medications, buy a pill minder box at a drug store or pharmacy. Be sure the pill minder has the number of slots that you need. For example, if your loved one takes medications 4x/day, be sure the pill minder boxes have four slots per day. (Helpful hint: I purchased four of these boxes, each one lasting one week. Then my mother's pills are set up once a month.)

Typical Service Delivery Models: First, the home health nurse will contact you within one to two days after your loved one arrives home from rehab. The RN will come and do a home assessment where he/she will ask questions about what your love -one needs. Based on this assessment, the nurse determines if your loved one needs physical therapy, occupational therapy, speech therapy, and/or home health aide for showering and self-care.

Therapy Services in the Home: Home health therapy services were not intended to be intensive or daily rehabilitation. The occupational, physical, and/or speech therapist will come and perform an assessment. Based on the assessment, therapy services will be prescribed. In most cases, these will only be done 1–2x/week. The purpose of home health care therapies is to train you, the family, and the patient on how to carry through on home exercises.

Community Reintegration Services: Many cities have wonderful senior centers with activities daily at a minimal yearly cost. Take advantage of the exercise and craft classes many offers. In many cases, they also offer a free lunch service. Some senior centers will provide a van for transportation to and from the center.

Community Transportation Services: Many cities have free medical related transportation services for patients using a wheelchair. Double check with your city's transportation services as to what is available for people with disabilities as far as medical and nonmedical transportation. In many cases, a guest may ride with the person for a nominal fee.

Companion Services: These services are provided by private agencies on an hourly basis. In many cases, the patient does not need a medically trained professional to stay in the home with them but a companion to help with light housekeeping, meals, activities and transportation. Nonmedical companion services are much cheaper than medical home services. Companion services can run, in most cases, between $12–$15/hr. (prices vary from city to city). Skilled medical home services, especially nursing services, can run as high as $30/hr. Companions cannot administer medications in most cases. They can assist with showering/bathing, dressing, and other personal care activities.

NOTES

CHAPTER 7

FREQUENTLY ASKED QUESTIONS

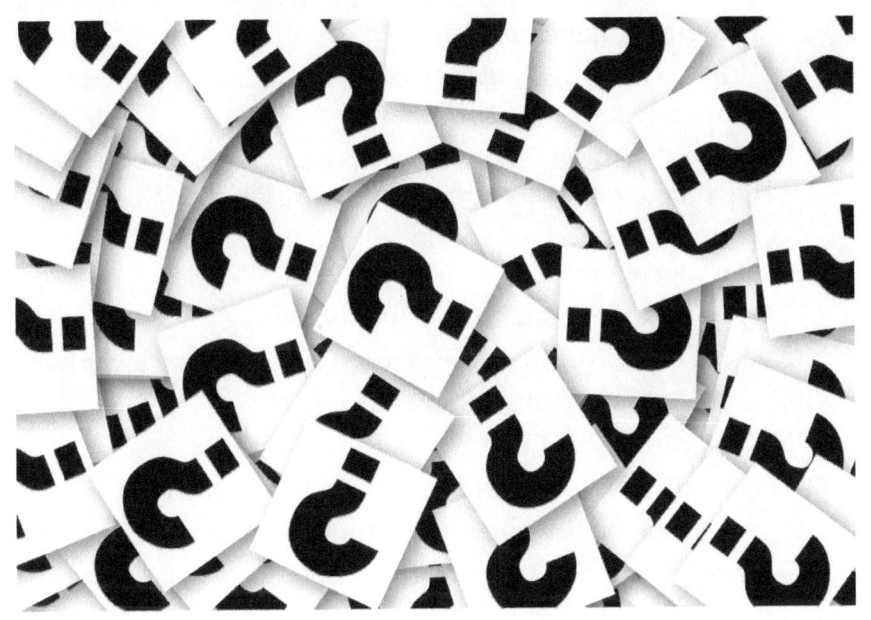

1) How long will my loved one be in rehab?
2) What therapies will my loved one receive while in rehab?
3) How many hours per day will my loved one receive therapy?
4) Will my loved one have the same therapists every day?
5) Who do I talk to about my loved one's therapy and progress?
6) When do I see the facility doctor, and how frequently will he/she see my loved one?
7) How will I get records of the rehab stay to show my loved one's primary care physician?
8) Do you need me to bring in my loved one's medications that they take at home regularly?
9) Who do I talk to about how much the insurance will pay and benefits to cover the rehab stay?
10) When do I meet with the therapists and staff to hear about the progress and discharge plan for my loved one?
11) How do I appeal a decision to discharge my loved one if I don't agree with it?
12) How do I report an issue or file a grievance?
13) What is involved in getting a private room for my loved one?
14) Can I stay overnight with my loved one?
15) When are visiting hours?
16) How many visitors can come to see my loved one?
17) When are the best times to visit my loved one?
18) When are meal times, and can I join my loved one for meals? How do I do this?
19) Who will do my loved one's laundry while he/she is in the rehab facility?
20) Should I label all of my loved one's personal items and clothes?
21) Can I bring in food or special items for my loved one?

22) Who do I talk with about the activity programs, and how do I know when activities are scheduled that might interest my loved one?

23) How many days before discharge will I be informed about the discharge date?

24) Who will order the equipment my loved one needs for home? Will the insurance pay for durable medical equipment (i.e. bathroom equipment, W/C, etc.)?

25) When will the rehab staff train the family on what the patient needs, so the family can help them at home?

26) How do I get my loved one's wound care supplies? Will the home health care nurse provide these? What about diapers/ briefs? Are these covered by insurance, or does the family need to buy them?

27) What about tube feedings? Will the family be trained on how to do these feedings? Who will supply the tube feeding formula? Is this covered by insurance?

28) Who can provide us (the family) with a list of home health and companion services agencies?

29) Will my loved one have a home exercise program? Who provides this? Will we be trained on the program before discharge?

30) Are there religious services available for my loved one while they are here?

NOTES

CHAPTER 8

ORGANIZATIONS AND ONLINE RESOURCES

(Some of these are also present in my first book)

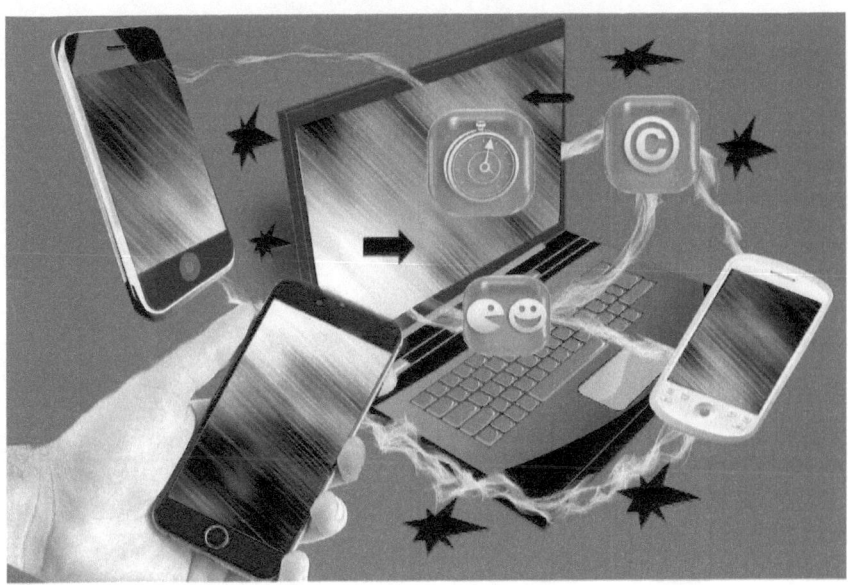

Alzheimer's Disease and Dementia

Alzheimer's Disease defined:

Dementia Types and Definitions:

One of the best and most insightful articles I have ever read regarding dementia from the perspective of a Caregiver is "The Deviousness of Dementia" by Dasha Kiper for the *American Scholar* magazine. I have provided the link here:

http://www.theguardian.com/society/2015/oct/20/the-deviousness-of-dementia?CMP=share_btn_fb

Elderly Services

Department of Health and Human Services Office of Senior Affairs
www.hhs.gov

National Organizations

Brain Injury Association of America, Inc.

1608 Spring Hill Rd
Suite 110
Vienna, VA 22182
braininjuryinfo@biausa.org
http://www.biausa.org 🖗
Tel: 703-761-0750 800-444-6443
Fax: 703-761-0755

Family Caregiver Alliance/National Center on Caregiving

785 Market St.
Suite 750
San Francisco, CA 94103
info@caregiver.org
http://www.caregiver.org 🖗
Tel: 415-434-3388 800-445-8106
Fax: 415-434-3508

National Alliance for Caregiving
4720 Montgomery Lane, 2nd Floor
Bethesda, MD 20814
(301) 718-8444 PH
(301) 951-9067 FAX
info@caregiving.org

National Association of State Head injury Administrators
(800)444-6443
www.nashia.org

National Rehabilitation Information Center (NARIC)
8201 Corporate Drive
Suite 600
Landover, MD 20785
naricinfo@heitechservices.com
http://www.naric.com 🔗
Tel: 301-459-5900/301-459-5984 (TTY) 800-346-2742
Fax: 301-562-2401

National Stroke Association
9707 E. Easter lane
Englewood, CO 80112
(303) 649-9299 (800) 787-6537
www.stroke.org

National Spinal Cord Injury Association
6701 Democracy Blvd Suite 300-9
Bethesda, MD 20817
www.spinaldord.org

National Center on Shaken Baby Syndrome
2955 Harrison Blvd Suite 102
Ogden, UT 84403
★801) 627-3399 (888) 273-0071
www.dontshake.com

Helpful Websites

Traumatic Brain Injury-Resources for Veterans with TBI
www.maketheconnection.net/TBI

Medical Equipment Information:
http://www.medicare.gov/what-medicare-covers/part-b/durable-medical-equipment.html

Head Trauma Resource-BrainInjury.com
www.**braininjury**.com

The Brain Trauma Foundation
https://www.**brain**trauma.org/

Brain Injury Association of America
www.biausa.org/

National Institute of Neurological Disorders and Stroke
http://www.ninds.nih.gov/disorders/tbi/org_tbi.htm

The National Parkinson's Association
www.parkinsons.org

Alzheimer's and Dementia Foundation/Association
www.alz.org

Centers for Medicare and Medicaid
www.mymedicareanswers.com

NOTES

CHAPTER 9

HOME EXERCISE SUGGESTIONS

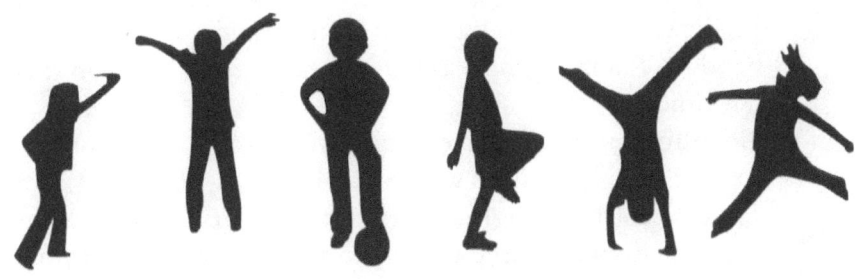

Respiratory Exercises to Improve Lung Function

Do these exercises two to three times per day. It may be helpful to remember to do them after breakfast, after lunch, and after dinner. Sit unsupported in your W/C (do not lean back against the backrest) or at the edge of your bed with feet planted firmly on the floor.

1) Sit upright and raise the chest. Press the shoulder blades together. Reach up to the slowly ceiling as high as you can. As you do this, inhale deeply, feeling the bottom part of your lungs expand. Lower arms to a long exhale. Do this ten times.

2) Place your hands over your abdomen. As you inhale, push out your hands to expand the lower part of your lungs. Inhale to the slow count of ten. Exhale and push with your hands to forcibly exhale as fast and hard as you can. Do this ten times.

3) Coughing practice: Place your hands over your abdomen. As you cough, pull in with your hands as forcibly as you can to assist the cough and strengthen it. Try to cough up any secretions and keep pulling in your abdomen with your hands as you cough to strengthen the cough. Do this ten times

4) Incentive Spirometer (IS): First, turn your head away from the IS and blow forcibly like you are blowing out a candle placed three feet away. Then, when you have expelled all the air from your lungs, place your mouth over the mouthpiece and inhale, long and slowly, making the white or blue disc in the middle rise slowly toward your goal. At the same time, the "helicopter" on the side must rise slowly and hover between the good and best marks on some devices or between the arrows on others. Both things are equally important. Long and slow inhale. Long and prolonged as best you can. Be sure to check your posture during these exercises. The chest should be lifted with as much space as you can get between the bottom of your last rib and your pelvis. Do these ten times.

All of the above exercises will make you cough. This demonstrates that you are moving air more, and now may be able to cough up any infectious secretions that have taken up residence in your long bases. Remember, posture is the key to success. Raise the chest and try to sit as tall as you possibly can. Try to repeat these exercises 2x/day. Then build up to 3x/day. For any questions, please contact me or any other occupational therapist. Feel free to show them this list, and keep it handy on your tray table to use daily.

Bed Exercises

1) With knee straight and ankle on top of a rolled up towel, push the back of the knee into the bed and hold for five seconds. Repeat ten times. Do three sets.
2) With knee extended, slide the heel up toward your bottom, bending the knee to ninety degrees or as much as possible. Slide the foot back down to straighten the knee. Do this ten times. Do three sets.
3) With knee straight, raise the leg of the bed about six inches and hold to a slow count of five. Then lower the leg back down to the bed. Repeat ten times. Do three sets.
4) Sit up in the wheelchair. Place a towel under your foot and "clean the floor." Do this for ten minutes.
5) Sit up in the wheelchair. March your feet while sitting, lifting knees up as high as possible. Repeat ten times. Do three sets
6) Sit up in the wheelchair and kick each foot out in front of you, alternating the feet. Repeat ten times. Do three sets.
7) Propel your wheelchair without using your arms. Use your feet only.

Sternal Precautions After Open Chest Surgery
Melanie M. Tidman DHSc, MA, OTR/L

Your doctor should have provided a list of precautions for you to follow as your chest heals. This healing process may take up to 6-8 weeks. You will need to carefully monitor your arm movements to insure your chest heals properly. If you feel pain at the incision site or in the middle of your chest, stop what you are doing. The following are some suggestions to follow once you get home:

1) When getting out of bed, roll to your side, cross one arm across your chest and using your stomach muscles come up to sit at the edge of the bed only using the arm opposite the side you are laying on to gently push up to sit. Use your pushing arm 20% and your stomach and back muscles 80%.

2) When coming up to standing, do not push with both arms, use your legs. When moving, it is a good idea to cross your arms across your chest.

3) When raising your arms, do not go higher than your shoulder height.

4) Take care not to bring your arms back behind your body with opening the chest which might put strain on the healing incision. Most of your movements will be forward and across your body.

5) Do not lift anything more than a gallon of milk (approx. 8-10lbs).

6) Do not push or pull with your arms (i.e. grabbing a bar and pulling yourself up to stand)

7) When getting back into bed, sit on the edge of the bed, lower yourself to your side not using your arms, bend your knees and bring them up onto the bed, roll onto your back. Repeat the process in reverse order to come up to sit at the edge of the bed.

8) You can reach up to brush or wash your hair. Just use one hand at a time. When in doubt, cross the other arm across your chest for protection during any movement with one arm/hand.

9) When dressing, be sure most movements are forward and you may dress normally. Pulling up pants is fine if they are lightweight and loose fitting. The same holds true with pulling pants down for toileting. Reaching down to your feet is permitted.

10) It will be very hard to get up from sitting if you are sitting on a low surface. Raise the level of the surfaces you sit on (you may have someone put blocks under a chair or couch) for ease of coming up to stand without using your arms.

11) Ask your doctor when you can shower.

12) Ask your doctor when you may drive

13) When sitting down in a chair, first back up to the chair so you can feel the chair behind BOTH legs. Then lower yourself with your legs. Crossing your arms across your chest will prevent you from pushing up or lowering using your arm strength.

14) Sitting down in the shower or tub is the safest way to bathe. A Tub Transfer bench for tub showers prevents you having to step into and out of the tub.

Remember, if the incision starts to drain, becomes red or inflamed, or opens in any way, contact your doctor immediately!

CHAPTER 10

GUIDELINES AND PRECAUTIONS

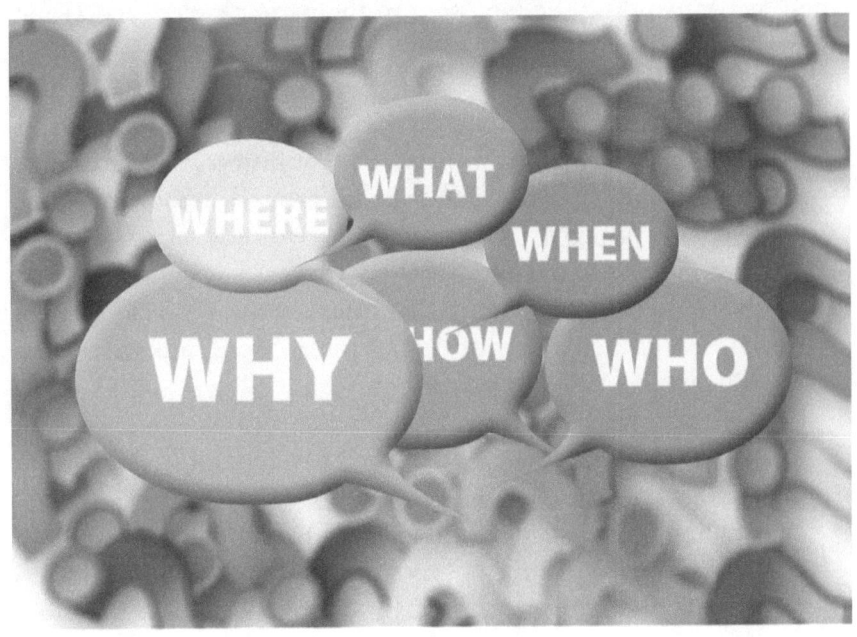

General Guidelines for Determining if Patients
Qualify for Skilled Rehabilitation

For Complete Guidelines go to www.cms.gov

Summary of Main Guidelines:

When leaving the hospital, there are general criteria that qualify a patient for skilled intervention in a skilled nursing facility rehabilitation center that doctors and therapists consider when recommending the next step in the patient's recovery. Good questions to ask include:

- Impairments and functional limitations in muscle performance (strength), joint mobility/ROM, motor function and control, gait, balance, arousal, aerobic capacity, and skin integrity or presence of wounds *and* deficits in motor control, strength, sensory processing, cognition, and psychological well-being that affect self-care performance, household management, social interaction, and safety that warrant PT/OT intervention.
- Unstable vital signs (i.e. blood pressure, heart rate, oxygen saturations) with activity that need to be monitored to ensure patient's safety.
- Bracing, splinting, or casting needs in addition to any assistive devices or environmental modification needs.
- Need for caregiver training (range of motion, positioning, skin checks for skin integrity, wound care or dressing changes, assisting ambulation and self-care tasks, donning slings, orthotics, etc.)
- Patient's education (precautions, techniques to enhance walking or general movement, energy conservation concepts, use of adaptive equipment, and environmental modifications)

If general criteria show *non-readiness* for skilled intervention and the patient needs a lower frequency/intensity/duration of skilled intervention:

- Rancho Los Amigos Scale I or II with minimal or no response to therapeutic intervention
- Medically fragile or unstable unless cleared for mobility by MD or lead PT/OT
- On CAGE protocol (withdrawing from alcohol toxicity) and unable to appropriately establish patient's functional level 2/2 medications influence on mobility or completion of self-care
- Sedated on a ventilator and unable to actively participate in therapy interventions
- All criteria for skilled intervention above—particularly with respect to family training—have been met.
- Severe cognitive limitations, combative behaviors, or refuses treatment

Or if the patient does not need skilled rehabilitation, the patient may meet the following:

- Patient is independent for functional mobility and completion of self-care but may only need assistance for lines or equipment management to engage in mobility, ambulation, supervision, or minimal assistance for basic self-care tasks such as toileting, bathing, dressing, meal preparation, transportation, or mobility with assistive devices (i.e. walker or cane).

How to decide whether your loved one needs acute rehabilitation (three to five hours of therapy daily) or skilled rehabilitation (two to three hours of therapy daily):

My rule of thumb after thirty-eight years of practice includes the following questions:

- Is patient over the age of seventy-five?
- Is patient able to tolerate up to five hours of therapy per day?
- Is patient able to follow verbal instructions?

- Is patient able to remember verbal instructions and safety instructions?
- Is patient able and willing to participate?
- Is the goal to transition patient back to their home?
- Does the patient live alone?
- Will the patient have assistance available 24/7 once discharged?

Concepts to keep in mind when helping your loved one to adjust to being at home:

1. Simplify the task
2. Allow extra time
3. Establish a simple routine
4. Set out and arrange needed items
5. Break down the task into smaller parts
6. Label drawers, containers, or cabinets

Family Interventions for Patients with Cognitive Deficits: (Rancho Los Amigos Scale, see www.neuroskills.com/resources/**rancho-los-amigos**-revised.php)

Cognitive Level 1–3

- Explain to the individual what you are about to do For example, "I'm going to move your leg."
- Talk in a normal tone of voice.
- Keep comments and questions short and simple. For example, instead of "Can you turn your head to look at me," direct them to "Look at me."

Cognitive Level 4

- Tell the person who you are, where he is, why he is there, and what day it is. May need to do this repeatedly
- Limit the number of visitors to two to three people at a time. Keep noise in the room low, speak in soft tones

O Keep the room calm and quiet. Provide frequent breaks in the action.
O Bring in favorite belongings and pictures of family members and close friends.
O Allow the person extra time to respond, but don't expect responses to be correct.
O Sometimes the person may not respond at all.
O Give him rest periods. He will tire easily.
O Engage him in familiar activities, such as listening to his favorite music, talking about the family and friends, reading out loud to him, watching TV, combing his hair, putting on lotion, etc.

Cognitive Level 5

O Avoid playing into inappropriate behaviors
O Use redirection and distraction
O Do not try to reason with the person
O Assume short term memory deficits, use frequent repetition
O Keep comments short and simple
O Remind person of the day, date, name, location, and reason they are here
O Organize and simplify tasks
O Bring in family pictures and familiar objects
O Give frequent rest breaks

Cognitive Level 6

O Person is unaware of their deficits
O Don't argue with the person
O Encourage rehabilitation program participation
O Frequent repetition of instructions when needed
O Journal with the person on daily events
O Help to initiate activities through use of a written or pictorial schedule

Cognitive Level 7

- Treat person as their PLOF
- Try not to tease or use slang. Keep it simple
- Reassure and discuss deficits
- Try to return to PLOF routines and activities
- Discuss emotions and coping strategies
- Seek outside support and counseling

(Note: These strategies also may work with patients with dementia or other cognitive symptoms.)

The Environmental Skill–Building Program for Caregivers
ESP is designed to provide family caregivers with

- Education about the disease process and the impact of environments on care recipient behaviors
- Problem-solving techniques to identify antecedents and consequences of targeted problem behaviors, and
- Technical skills to modify the home.
- http://www.rosalynncarter.org/education_support/

REFERENCES

American Occupational Therapy Association—http://www.aota.org/

American Physical Therapy Association—http://www.apta.org/

American Speech and Hearing Association—http://www.asha.org

Caregiver Alliance—www.cargiverslibrary.com

Rancho Los Amigos Recovery Scale, retrieved from https://www. jhsmh.org/LinkClick.aspx?fileticket=8hAd-OqTIQ0%3D& tabid=298